医療職が覚えておきたい

運動・動作の英語表現

監修：柳澤　健（城西国際大学福祉総合学部教授・理学療法学科長）
著　：飯田恭子（首都大学東京名誉教授）

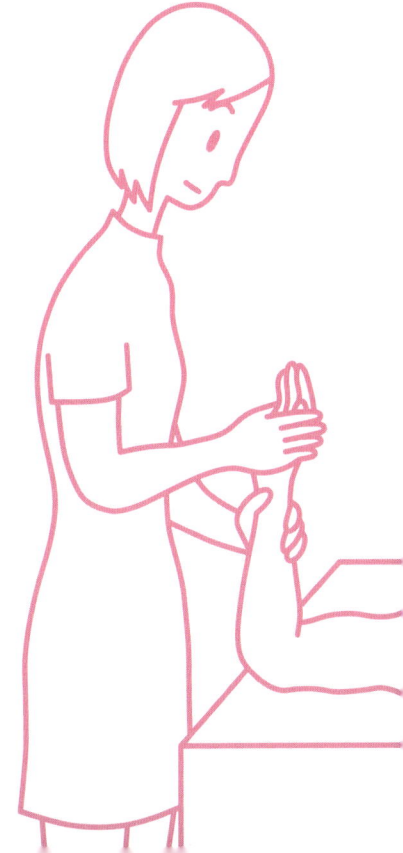

医学書院

医療職が覚えておきたい運動・動作の英語表現

発　行	2007年5月15日　第1版第1刷Ⓒ
	2017年10月15日　第1版第7刷

監　修　柳澤　健
　　　　やなぎさわ　けん

著　者　飯田恭子
　　　　いいだ やすこ

発行者　株式会社　医学書院
　　　　代表取締役　金原　優
　　　　〒113-8719　東京都文京区本郷 1-28-23
　　　　電話　03-3817-5600(社内案内)

印刷・製本　山口北州印刷

本書の複製権・翻訳権・上映権・譲渡権・貸与権・公衆送信権(送信可能化権を含む)は株式会社医学書院が保有します.

ISBN978-4-260-00389-6

本書を無断で複製する行為(複写, スキャン, デジタルデータ化など)は,「私的使用のための複製」など著作権法上の限られた例外を除き禁じられています. 大学, 病院, 診療所, 企業などにおいて, 業務上使用する目的(診療, 研究活動を含む)で上記の行為を行うことは, その使用範囲が内部的であっても, 私的使用には該当せず, 違法です. また私的使用に該当する場合であっても, 代行業者等の第三者に依頼して上記の行為を行うことは違法となります.

JCOPY 〈出版者著作権管理機構　委託出版物〉
本書の無断複製は著作権法上での例外を除き禁じられています.
複製される場合は, そのつど事前に, 出版者著作権管理機構
(電話 03-3513-6969, FAX 03-3513-6979, info@jcopy.or.jp)の
許諾を得てください.

はじめに

　高齢社会を豊かで実りあるものにするためには、一人でも多くの人が何らかの病気や障害をもちながらも社会の中の一員として身体的・精神的に元気に活動していけるようなシステム作りが大切です。そのために看護・医療・リハビリテーションの専門職たちの果たす役割は大きく、すぐれた指導や援助活動が期待されます。加齢や疾病・障害によって、しばしば一時的にまた進行的に全身の機能低下や障害が生じたり、また身体のさまざまな部位のmotion やmovement が妨げられたりすることは避けられないことです。しかし近年は、高度に進んだ専門的知識や技術によってこれまで以上に健康回復や自立性の回復への道が広がってきています。さまざまな身体的不都合を抱えながらも、可能な限り日常生活を積極的に維持し、活発な精神活動、仕事や余暇活動、コミュニティ活動など社会生活、経済生活を享受していけるよう、看護・医療そしてリハビリテーションの専門職は最先端の理論に裏付けられたスキルを駆使することによって、大切な役割を果たしていかねばなりません。

　精神的・身体的に機能が衰え、身体の動きがスムースにいかないクライエントに対するプロとしての指示や説明のことばや表現は、具体的でわかりやすく、詳細でありなが

らも効率よく、また解剖学的にも矛盾がなく、生理学的にも適正でなくてはなりません。しかし、筋骨格系、神経系はもちろんのこと、身体のあらゆる部位の動きについてのアセスメント、診断・治療、処置、ケア、日常生活、リハビリテーションを行う上での指示や説明の用語や表現は案外と難しく、英語はもちろんのこと日本語においても具体的な例示はほとんど見あたりません。

　本書では、起きてから寝るまでの日常生活動作、運動・動作表現、診断・機能評価の表現、治療上の体位の表現、訓練・リハビリテーションの表現などについて、クライエントつまり素人向けへの指示や説明の文を専門の表現と対比しながら平易な英文で作成してあります。なお、運動・動作の表現については、首都大学東京の柳澤健教授にご専門の立場からご指導いただきました。

　国内外における、外国人患者への対応時にまた、専門職としての語学力のスキルアップに使っていただければ幸いです。

著者　飯田恭子

CONTENTS

PART 1　起きてから寝るまでの日常生活動作表現

section 1	Waking up	起きる	008
section 2	At the bathroom	歯磨き・洗顔をする	010
section 3	Brushing up	髪をとかす	014
section 4	Getting dressed	着がえる	016
section 5	Toileting	トイレに行く	020
section 6	Eating	食べる	022
section 7	Making tea	お茶を入れる	024
section 8	Transportation	外出する	026
section 9	Housekeeping	家事をする	028
section 10	Recreation	余暇を楽しむ	030
section 11	Having a bath	お風呂に入る	032
section 12	Bedtime	寝る	034

CONTENTS

PART 2　病院の中での運動・動作表現

section 1　Physical Exercise:Lying Position　　038
　　　　　　体操の表現：マット上で

section 2　Physical Exercise:Sitting Position　　043
　　　　　　体操の表現：椅子を使って

section 3　Physical Exercise:Standing Position　046
　　　　　　体操の表現：立位で

section 4　Passive ROM Exercise　　050
　　　　　　他動的関節可動域訓練

section 5　Muscle Test:Upper Body　　052
　　　　　　筋力測定評価：上半身

section 6　Muscle Test:Lower Body　　059
　　　　　　筋力測定評価：下半身

section 7　Functional Assessments　　062
　　　　　　さまざまな機能検査

section 8　Diagnostic Tests　　070
　　　　　　さまざまな診断検査

section 9　Positioning　　076
　　　　　　体位

付録：関節可動域運動の専門的な表現と一般的な表現　　083

PART 1

起きてから寝るまでの日常生活動作表現

section 1 Waking up
起きる

Pull the coverlet to one side.
  掛け布団をとる

Stretch your arms above your head.
  両腕を頭の上に伸ばす

Stretch your legs.
  両脚を伸ばす

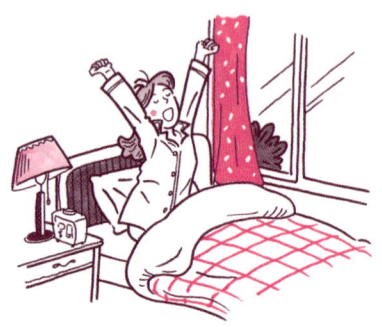

Raise yourself on one elbow.
  片肘をついて体を起こす

Roll your head in a circle clockwise and counterclockwise.
  首を時計回りと反時計回りに回す

Tilt your head side to side.
  首を左右に傾ける

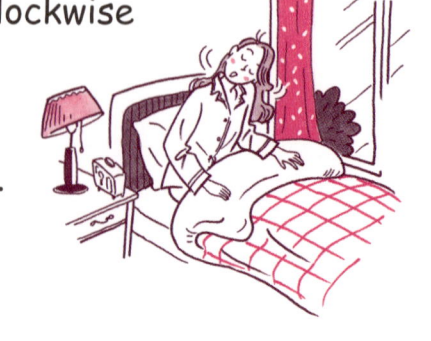

Rock your head forward.
Rock your head backward.
　首を前に傾ける。首を後ろにそらす

Swing both legs over the side of the bed.
　両脚をベッドサイドに振り下ろす

Sit at the edge of the bed.
　ベッドの端に座る

Press your palms against the bed,
while coming to a standing position.
　掌でベッドを押して立ち上がる

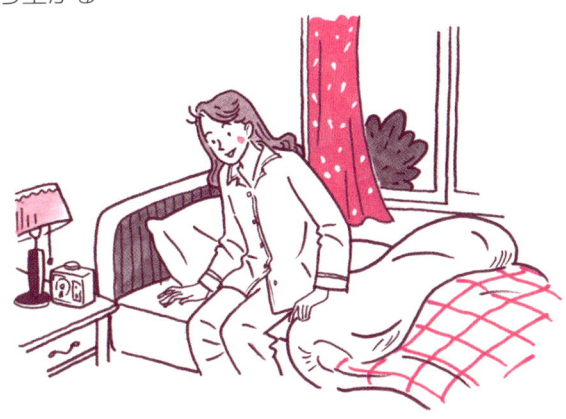

section 2 At the bathroom
歯磨き・洗顔をする

Roll up your sleeves.
　両腕をまくる
（参考）Bare your arms. ともいう。

Bend your upper body forward.
　上半身を前方に傾ける

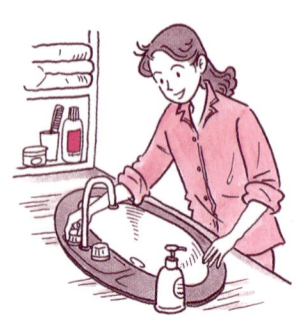

Turn on the tap of the faucet.
　蛇口をひねる

Rub your hands together under the running water.
　流水の下で手をこする

Press the decanter of the liquid soap.
　液体せっけんの栓を押す

Lather some soap in your hand.
　せっけんを泡立てる

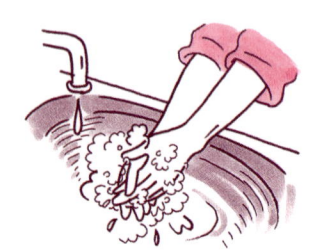

Wash the palms and the backs.
Wash between fingers.
　掌と手の甲を洗う。指の間を洗う

Massage gently your face with your soapy hands.
せっけんのついた手で顔をそっとなでる

Put your hands together under the running water.
両手で流水を受ける

Bring your hands with water to your face.
両手で水を顔に近づける

Rub your face softly with your hands.
両手で顔をやさしくこする

Rinse the soap off your face.
せっけんをすすぎ落とす

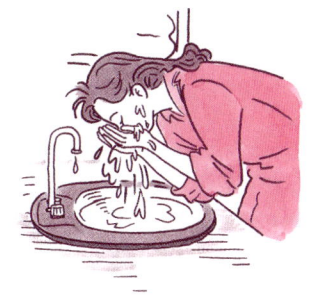

Take a towel and dry your hands and face.
タオルをとって手と顔を拭く

Hang the towel on a towel rack.
タオルをタオル掛けに掛ける

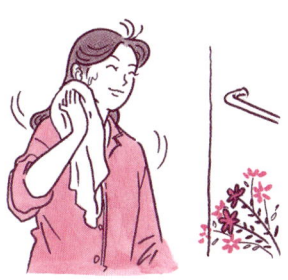

section2 At the bathroom　歯磨き・洗顔をする

Wrap your hand around the glass and grasp it firmly.
コップに手を回し、しっかり握る

Bring the cup to your mouth.
コップを口のところへもっていく

Fill your mouth partially with water without swallowing.
水を飲み込まず口に含む

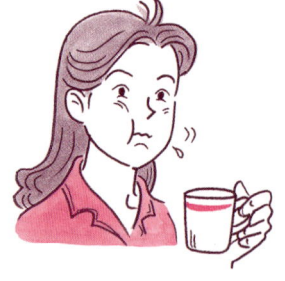

Rinse your mouth out.
口をすすぐ

Swish the water in your mouth.
口の中で水をクチュクチュとする

Spit out the water.
水を吐き出す

Put water into your mouth.
水を口に含む

Tilt your head backward and gargle your throat.
頭を後方に傾けてうがいをする

Pick up the toothbrush with your thumb and index finger.
親指と人差し指で歯ブラシを取り上げる

Support the toothbrush with your other fingers.
ほかの指で歯ブラシを支える

Pick up toothpaste with the opposite hand.
もう片方の手で歯磨き粉をとる

Remove the lid, squeeze the toothpaste onto the toothbrush.
蓋を開けて歯磨き粉を歯ブラシにつける

Brush your teeth up and down, back and forth.
上下左右に歯を磨く

Spit out the toothpaste and rinse out your mouth.
歯磨き粉を吐き出し、口をすすぐ

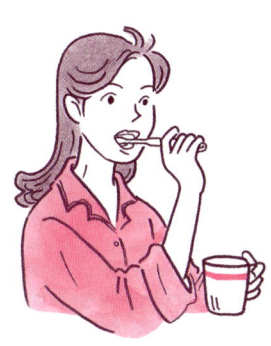

section 3 Brushing up
髪をとかす

Look at yourself in the mirror.
鏡を見る

Grasp the handle of the brush.
ブラシの柄を握る

Raise your elbow to shoulder height.
肘を肩の高さまで持ち上げる

Run a brush through your hair.
髪にブラシを流す

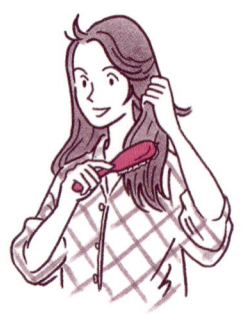

Comb your hair.
髪をくしでとかす

Run your hands through your hair.
両手で髪をかき上げる

Plug in the hair dryer.
ドライヤーのコンセントを入れる

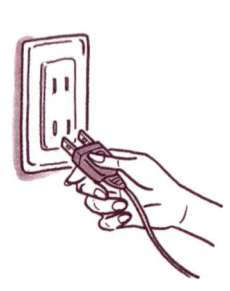

Dry your hair.
髪を乾かす

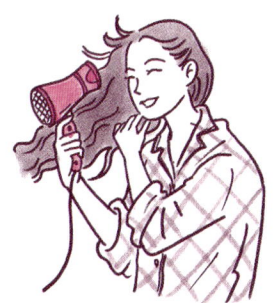

Bend your hands at the joints and run your fingers through your hair.
手の関節を曲げて、手櫛をする

Rub in hair cream with your fingertips.
ヘアクリームを指先ですりこむ

Press the nozzle to release spray.
ノズルを押してスプレーをかける

section 4 Getting dressed
着がえる

Put on a T-shirt.
　Tシャツを着る

Work your arms through the sleeves.
　袖に両腕を通す

Pull the T-shirt down over your head.
　Tシャツに頭を通す

Pull the bottom of your shirt down.
　シャツの裾を引き下げる

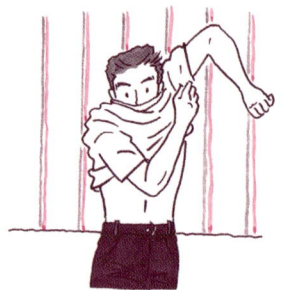

Put on a white shirt.
　ワイシャツを着る

Grasp the front of the shirt with one hand and put your opposite hand into the sleeve.
　シャツの前部分を持って、片方の腕を通す

Reach behind your back with the free arm and slip your arm into the sleeve.
　空いた手で後ろ手にシャツをつかんで、袖を通す

Swing your arm out.
腕を通す

Button a shirt.
シャツのボタンをはめる

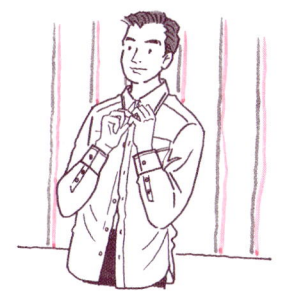

Push the button through the hole with the thumb and forefinger of one hand.
片手の親指と人差し指でボタンの穴にボタンを通す

Button the shirt from the top to down.
上から下へとボタンをとめていく

Put on a pair of pants.
ズボンをはく

Step into one pant leg.
ズボンの片脚に足を通す

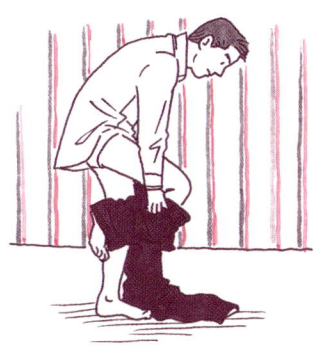

Then, step into the other.
もう片方の足も通す

Pull the pants up.
ズボンを引き上げる

section4 Gettnig dressed 着がえる

Put on your socks.
靴下をはく

Sit on the chair and raise one leg with bent knee.
椅子に座って、膝を曲げたまま片脚を上げる

Cross your leg over the opposite thigh.
その足を反対側の太腿の上に交差するようにのせる

Take one sock, and stretch it open with both hands.
片方の靴下を持って、両手で広げる

Insert your foot into the sock.
靴下の中に足を入れる

Pull it over your heel and up over your ankle.
踵のところまで、さらにくるぶしまで靴下を引き上げる

Uncross your leg and set your foot back on the floor.
組んだ脚を元に戻し、床の上に足を下ろす

Do the same with your other leg.
もう一方の脚も同様にする

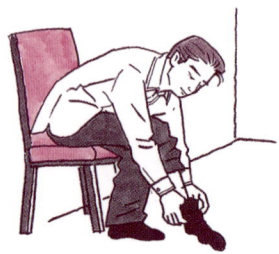

Zip up. (Unzip.)
ファスナーを上げる（下げる）

Hook up a dress. (Unhook a dress.)
ホックをとめる（はずす）

Tie your necktie. (Undo your necktie.)
ネクタイをしめる（ネクタイをはずす）

Wear a scarf around your neck. (Remove your scarf.)
スカーフを巻く（スカーフをとる）

Put on your coat.
コートをはおる

Take off your coat.
コートを脱ぐ

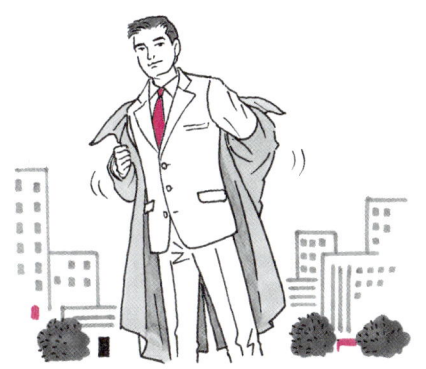

Put on your hat.
帽子をかぶる

Take off your hat.
帽子をとる

section 5 Toileting
トイレに行く

Enter the bathroom.
トイレに入る

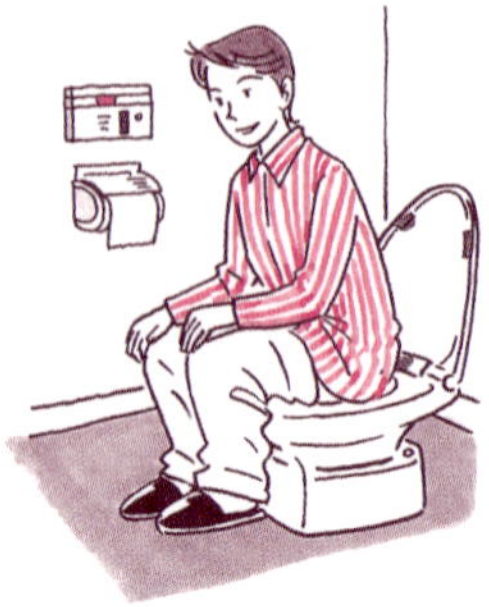

Pull down your over and under pants.
ズボンと下着のパンツを下ろす

Sit down on the toilet seat.
便座に腰をおろす

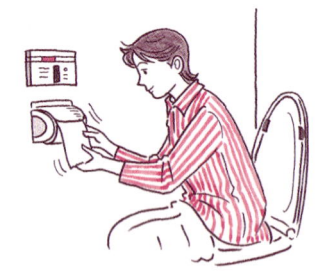

Set your bottom centered on the seat.
便座の中央におしりをおく

Press the button to wash your bottom.
ボタンを押しておしりを洗浄する

Take some toilet tissue and completely wipe your bottom.
トイレットペーパーをちぎっておしりをきれいに拭く

Stand up slowly and close the toilet lid.
ゆっくり立ち上がってトイレの蓋をする

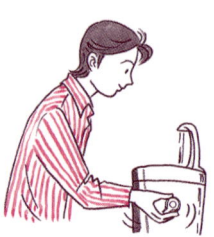

Flush the toilet.
水を流す

介助する場合の声かけ

Grasp the handrail and slowly approach the toilet seat.
手すりを持ってゆっくり便座に近づいてください

Put your weight bearing equally on both feet.
両足に均等に体重をかけてください

Attempt to sit on the toilet seat, while I am holding you around the waist.
胴体を抱えて支えていますから、便座に座ってみてください

Don't bear down and hold your breath while passing a stool.
排便時に力んだり、息を止めないでください

section 6 Eating
食べる

Clean your hands with a wet towel.
おしぼりで手を拭く

Pick up some of the food with the utensil.
ナイフとフォークで食べ物を取り上げる

Move the food to your mouth.
食べ物を口にもっていく

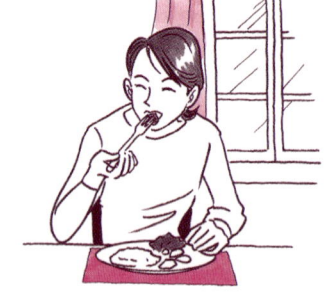

Masticate your food.
食べ物を咀嚼する

Swallow food.
食べ物を飲み込む

I have a fish bone stuck in my throat.
魚の骨がのどにつかえる

I choked on the tea.
お茶を飲んでむせる

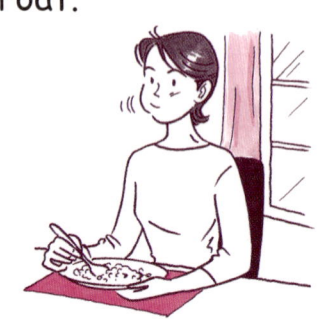

Wrap your hand around the glass.
コップに手を回してつかむ

Wrap both hands around the cup.
両手でコップを包んで持ち上げる

Bring a cup to your mouth.
コップを口にもっていく

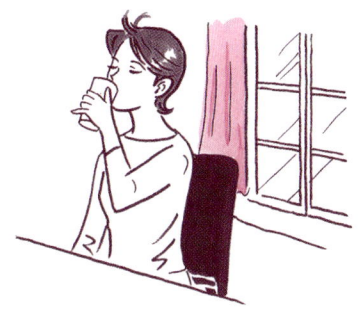

Scoop the soup with the spoon.
スプーンでスープをすくう

(参考) Eat your soup with a spoon.　eatを使ってスープを食することを表す。drinkは使わない

Mix the fruit into the yogurt with a spoon.
スプーンで果物とヨーグルトを混ぜ合わせる

Tear off small pieces of the bread.
パンを小さくちぎる

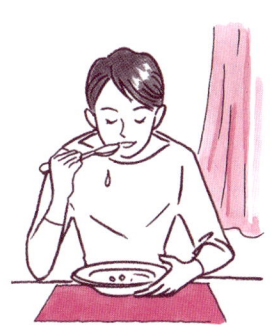

section 7 Making tea
お茶を入れる

Take a kettle and remove the lid from it.
　やかんをとって、蓋をとる

Fill the kettle with some water, and close the lid.
　やかんに水を入れて蓋をする

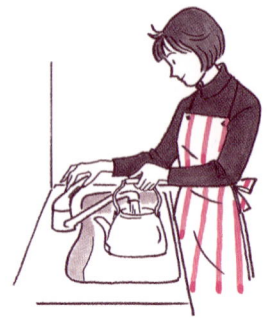

Grasp the handle and place it on the electric range.
　取っ手を握って電熱器の上にのせる
（参考）ガス台の場合は、gasring または、burner という

Wait for the water to boil.
　お湯が沸くまで待つ

Carefully grasp the handle and slowly pour boiling water into the teapot.
　気をつけて取っ手を握り、ゆっくりと
　ティポットにお湯を注ぐ

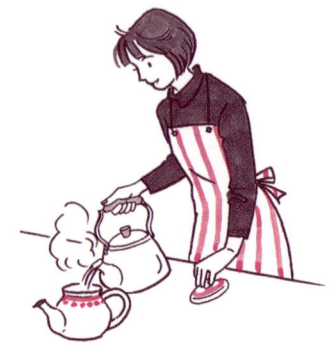

Tea leaves soak in hot water.
茶葉が湯につかる

Wait a couple of minutes for the leaves to soften.
茶葉がやわらかくなるまで2〜3分待つ

Strain the tea with a strainer.
お茶をこす

Pour the tea into the cup.
カップにお茶を注ぐ

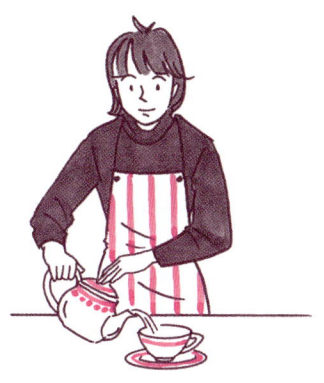

section 8 Transportation
外出する

Raise your arm straight up to hail a taxi.
まっすぐ手を上げてタクシーを呼ぶ

Take a taxi.
タクシーに乗る
(参考) takeは「乗って行く」という意味。
「乗り込む」は Get into the taxi.

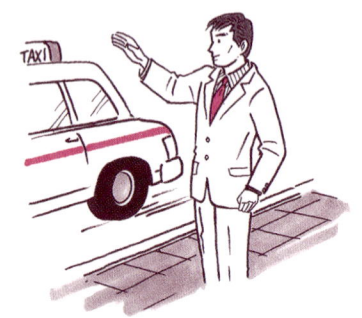

Take a train / a street car.
電車 / 路面電車に乗る

(参考)「乗り込む」は Board the train.

Take a seat.
シートに座る

Hold onto a strap.
つり革をつかむ

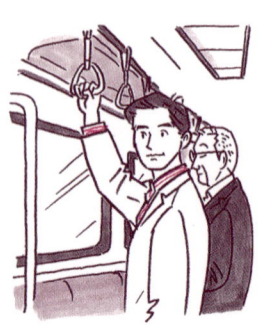

Climb / Go up the stairs.
階段を上がる

Go down the stairs.
階段を下りる

Go through the automated ticket barrier.
自動改札を抜ける

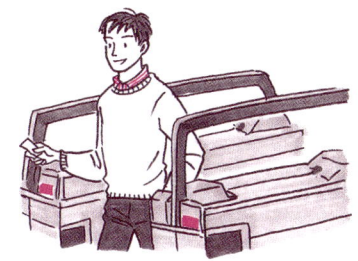

Ride a bicycle.
自転車に乗る

Pedal your bicycle.
ペダルをこぐ

Put your items in the basket.
荷物をかごに入れる

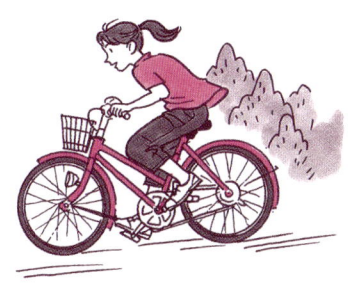

Drive a car.
車を運転する

Keep your things in the trunk of the car.
荷物を車のトランクに入れる

section 9 Housekeeping
家事をする

Run a vacuum cleaner in the room.
掃除機をかける

Squeeze the mop dry.
雑巾を絞る

Mop the floor.
雑巾で床を拭く

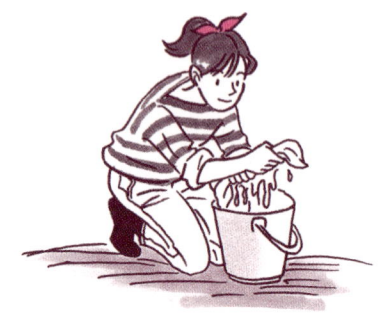

Do the laundry.
洗濯をする

(参考)「手洗いする」場合は、Do the laundry by hand.

Dry the wet clothes in the sun.
衣類を干す

Fold the laundry.
衣類をたたむ

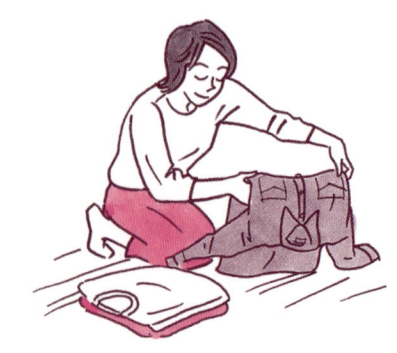

PART 1　起きてから寝るまでの日常生活動作表現

Do the cooking.
料理をする

Chop the vegetables with a kitchen knife.
野菜を包丁で切る

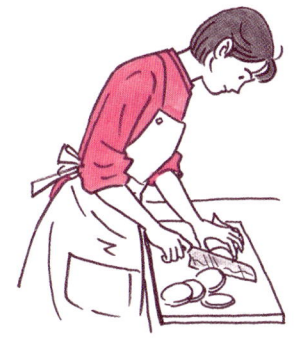

Fry foods in a frying pan. / Pantry the foods.
フライパンで炒める

Boil the potatoes.
ジャガイモをゆでる

Cook the root vegetables.
根菜類を煮る

Transfer the food to the plates.
料理を皿に盛る

section 10 Recreation
余暇を楽しむ

Read books and magazines.
読書をする

Turn each page.
ページをめくる

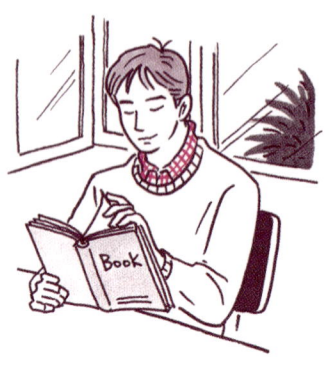

Listen to the music.
音楽を聴く

Watch the TV (program).
テレビを見る

Stroke the cat.
猫をなでる

Feed the dog.
犬にえさをやる

Walk the dog.
犬の散歩をする

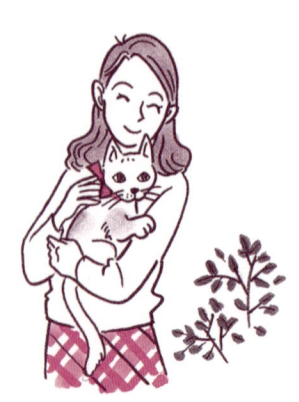

Water the plants.
植木に水をやる

Transfer the plant to a new pot.
植え替えをする

Add the fertilizer.
肥料をやる

Dig the soil with a hand shovel.
スコップで土を掘る

Plant the seeds.
種をまく

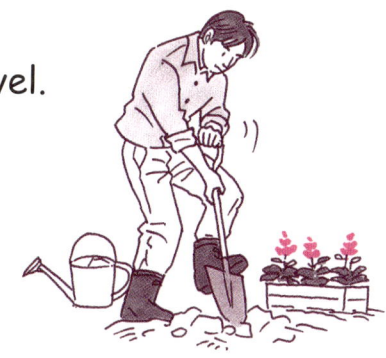

section 11 Having a bath
お風呂に入る

Take a shower.
シャワーを浴びる

Check the water temperature.
湯加減をみる

Enter the bath tub.
浴槽に入る

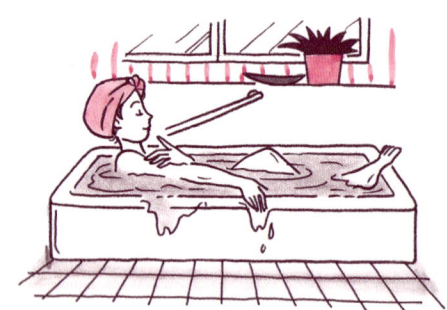

Wash your hair.
髪を洗う

Lean forward and rinse the shampoo from your hair.
前かがみになってシャンプーを洗い流す

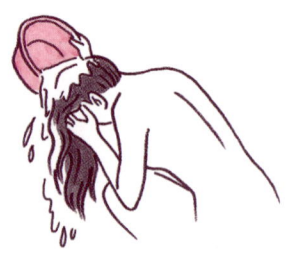

Lather the soap onto a wash cloth.
タオルでせっけんを泡立てる

Scrub your entire body from arm to foot.
腕から足まで体を洗う

Wash between your toes.
足の指の間まで洗う

Rinse the soap off your body.
せっけんを洗い流す

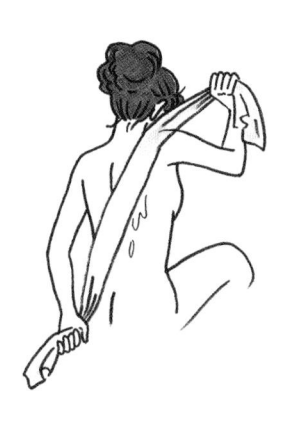

Dry your body with a towel.
タオルで体を拭く

Wrap a towel around your head.
頭にタオルを巻きつける

section 12 Bedtime
寝る

Yawn.
あくびをする

Rub your eyes.
目をこする

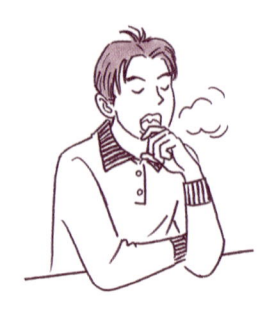

Put on your pajamas.
パジャマに着替える

Lie under the covers.
布団に入る

Turn off the light in the room.
部屋の明かりを消す

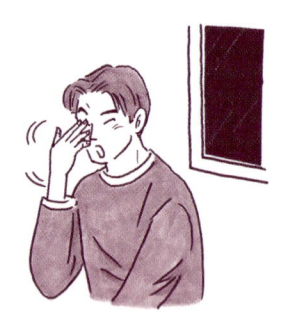

Go to sleep.
寝る

Snore.
いびきをかく

Grind your teeth.
歯ぎしりをする

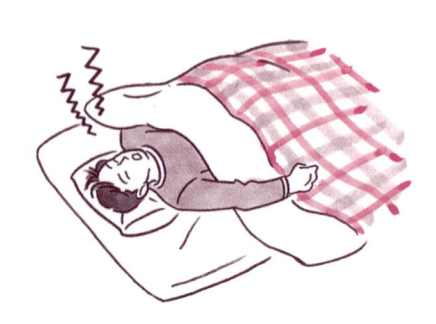

Talk in your sleep.
寝言を言う

Turn / Roll over in your bed.
寝返りをうつ

(参考) 眠れなくてゴロゴロと寝返りをうつ場合は、toss and turn という

PART 2

病院の中での運動・動作表現

section 1 Physical Exercise : Lying Position
体操の表現：マット上で

Lie on your back.
仰向けになる

Keep your back flat.
背中を平らにする

Legs elevated and close together.
両脚をぴったりくっつけて上げる

Elevate heels 3cm from the floor.
踵を床から3センチほど上げる

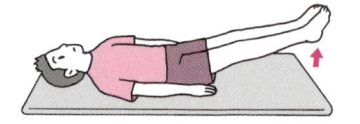

Pull your knees to your chest.
両膝を胸のほうに引っ張る

Curl your head up toward your knees.
頭を持ち上げ、両膝に近づける

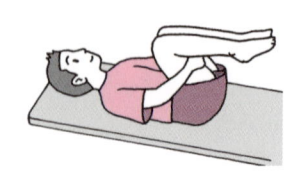

Bend one knee and gently pull it toward your chest.
片方の膝を曲げて、ゆっくり胸のほうに近づける

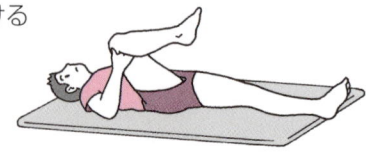

Right leg remains straight and flat on the floor.
　右脚は床の上にまっすぐに平らにしたままに
Bend your left knee at 90-degree.
　左の膝を90度に曲げる
Pull your knee across your body toward your opposite shoulder.
　膝を体の上で斜めに引き、反対側の肩に近づける

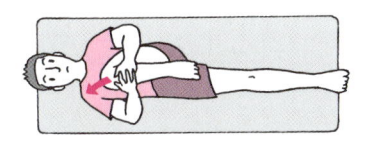

Bend your knees up on your back.
　仰向きになったまま膝を立てる
Let your knees fall apart.
　両膝を開いてパタンと落とす

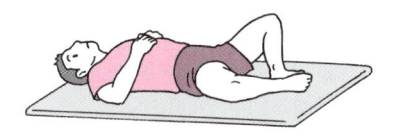

Bring your knees together.
　両膝をくっつける

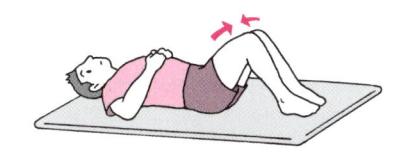

Bend both knees and roll over onto one side.
　両膝を曲げて、片側に転がる

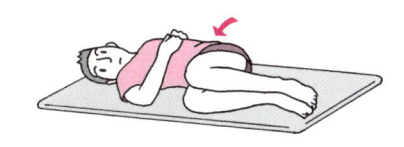

section1 Physical Exercise : Lying Position　体操の表現：マット上で

Spread your legs.
　　両脚を広げる
Lean forward from hips.
　　股関節のところから前にかがんでいく
Move your butt and hips forward.
　　お尻から股関節を前方に傾ける
Use hands for stability and support.
　　両手で支えて安定させる

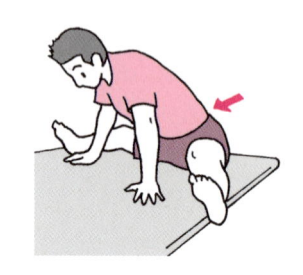

Spread your legs. Turn to face one foot.
　　両脚を広げ、片方の足に顔を向ける
Bend forward from the hips in that direction.
　　その方向に向けて股関節から前方に体を倒す
Hold your leg with hands at a point that gives you an ease stretch.
　　無理なく伸ばせるところで、足を両手でつかむ

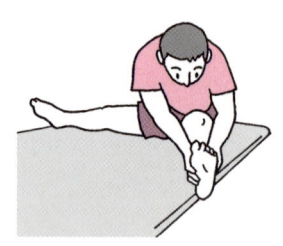

Lie on your stomach.
　　うつ伏せになる
Grasp your left foot with your left hand.
Heel touches the buttocks.
　　左手で左足をつかむ。踵はお尻に触れる

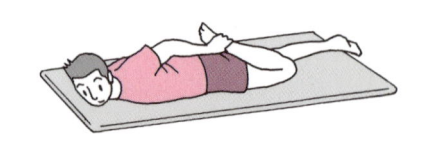

Front of the hips on the floor.
Elbows placed beneath your shoulder.
   腰の前側を床につける。両肘を両肩の下に置く
Extend your back upwards.
You feel a mild tension in your buttocks.
   背中を上方に伸ばす。お尻に少し力が入る

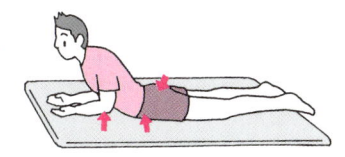

Sit with your legs bent under you.
   両脚を曲げて、その上に座る
Tops of your feet flat against the floor.
   両足の甲を床に平らにつける
Bend your torso onto your thighs.
   胴体を曲げて大腿の上におく
Reach forward with your hands.
   両手を前方に伸ばす

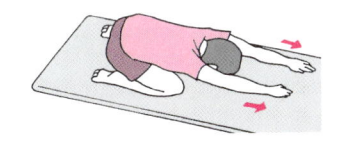

Get down on all fours.
   よつんばいになる
Support yourself on your hands and knees.
   両手と両膝で体を支える

Kneel down with palms on the floor
a comfortable distance from your knees.
   ひざまずいて両掌を膝の位置から適度に離して床につける
Lift your chin pulling your head back.
Expand your chest.
   あごを上げて頭を後ろにそらし、胸を張る

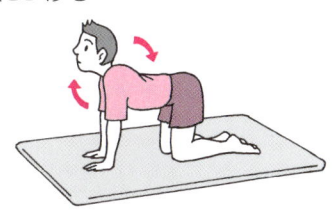

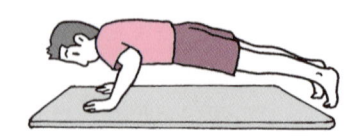

section1 Physical Exercise : Lying Position 体操の表現：マット上で

Lower your head.
Keep your neck and shoulder relaxed.
　頭を落とし、首と肩の力を抜く

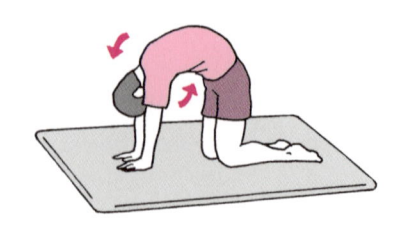

Do the push-ups.
　腕立て伏せをする
Lie on your stomach.
Palms on the floor with arms shoulder-width apart.
　うつ伏せになり、腕を肩幅に開いて、掌を床につける
Extend your arms and push your body up.
　両腕を伸ばし、体を押し上げる
Push your body down with an elbow angle of 90 degrees.
　両肘を直角に曲げて、体を押し下げる

section 2 Physical Exercise : Sitting Position
体操の表現：椅子を使って

Sit on a chair and lock your knees.
 椅子に座って膝を組む

Sit up on a chair. Extend your arms overhead.
 椅子にきちんと座って、両腕を頭上に伸ばす
Hold onto the outside of your left hand.
Pull your left arm to the side.
 左手の外側をつかみ、左腕を横に引っ張る

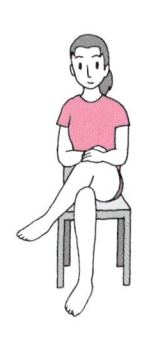

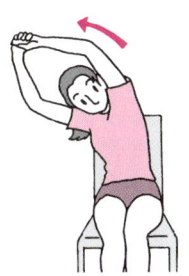

Sit on a chair and place the left ankle on the right knee.
 椅子に座り、左足首を右膝に乗せる
Rotate your ankles clockwise and then counter-clockwise.
 足首を時計回りにし、次に反時計回りに回す

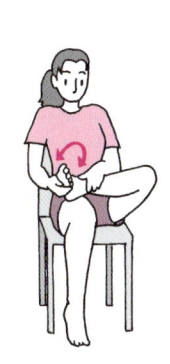

section2 Physical Exercise : Sitting Position　体操の表現：椅子を使って

Sit on a chair with both feet flat on the floor.
　椅子に座って両足を床に平らにつける
Lean forward to stretch your back placing your chest on your thighs.
　背中を伸ばして前傾姿勢になり、胸を大腿の上に置く
Keep palms on the floor.
　両掌を床につける

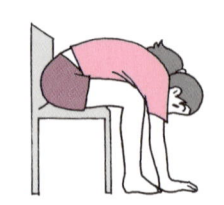

Keep your body aligned and use a chair for support. Rise onto the toes.
　体をまっすぐにして、椅子を支えにする。つま先立ちをする

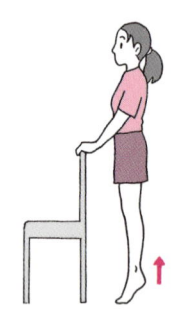

Sitting on a wheelchair, reach upward with one arm. Fingers extended.
　車椅子の上で、片腕を上方に伸ばす。手の指を伸ばして
Keep the other arm bent at the elbow.
Bend the torso slightly to the side.
　もう一方の腕は肘のところで曲げておく。
　胴体はやや横に曲げる

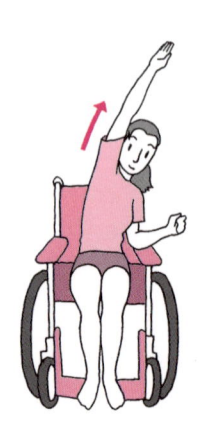

Sit up on the wheelchair.
Place a towel or strap around the ball of one foot.
　車椅子にきちんと座り、タオルか紐で片方の足の裏の
　ふくらみにあてる
Pull the strap(towel) toward the chest.
Extend the leg and strech your calf.
　紐（タオル）を自分の胸のほうに引く。
　脚を伸ばし、ふくらはぎのストレッチをする

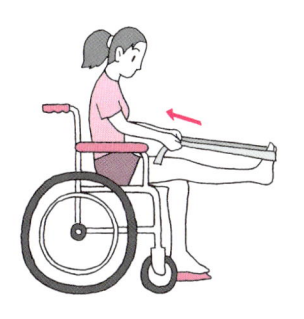

section 3 Physical Exercise : Standing Position
体操の表現：立位で

In a standing position, bend forward straightening your knees and touch your toes.
立位で膝を伸ばしたまま体を曲げてつま先に触れる

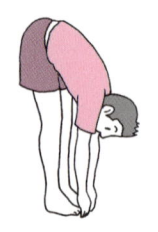

Alternate heel touches in front of the body.
体の前方へヒールタッチを交互に行う
（かかとを床につける動作）

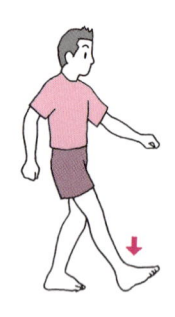

Your hands on your hips. Place the sole of the left foot against the inside of your right knee.
両手を腰にあてる。左の足裏を右膝の内側にあてる

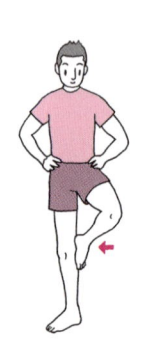

Stretch your arms out to the side.
Kick the right foot. Toe pointing downward, knees slightly bent.
   両腕を横に伸ばして、右足を蹴る。
   つま先を下に向け、膝は軽く曲げて

Swing arms in opposition to legs.
   腕と脚を逆に振る
Left arm is up when right knee is up.
   右膝が上がっているときは左腕が上がっている
Raise knee up parallel to the floor.
   膝を床に平行に上げる
Toes pointed down. Keep head up.
   つま先を下に向け、頭を上げて

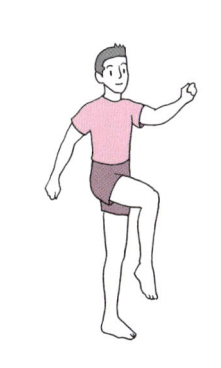

In a standing position, reach in opposite directions with both arms.
   立位になって、両腕を逆方向に伸ばす
Extend the left arm to overhead and the right one to the ground.
   左腕を頭上に伸ばし、右腕を地面のほうへ伸ばす

section3 Rhysical Exercise : Standing Position　体操の表現：立位で

Grasp your right hand with your left hand.
Extend both arms overhead.
　　左手で右手をつかむ。頭上で両腕を伸ばす
Pull the right arm over the head and down toward the ground. Bend slowly to the left.
　　右腕を頭の上で床方向に引っ張る。ゆっくり左側に曲げる

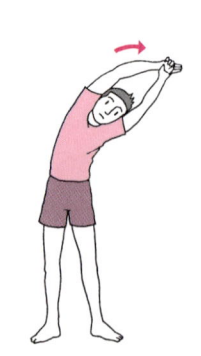

In a standing position, place one hand on your side for support.
　　立位になって、片手をわき腹のところにあてて支える
Extend arm up and over your head.
Bend at your waist to the side.
　　腕を頭上に上げて伸ばす。腰のところから横に曲げる
Your feet should be about shoulder-width apart.
Toes pointed outward.
　　両足はほぼ肩幅に開く。足の指は外側に向ける

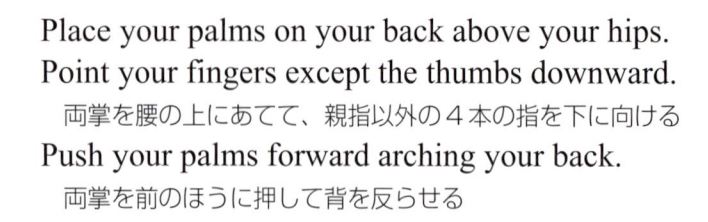

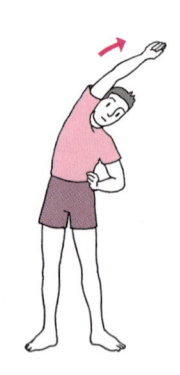

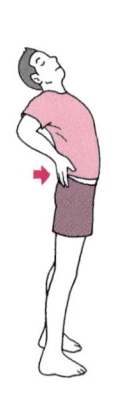

Place your palms on your back above your hips.
Point your fingers except the thumbs downward.
　　両掌を腰の上にあてて、親指以外の４本の指を下に向ける
Push your palms forward arching your back.
　　両掌を前のほうに押して背を反らせる

Raise the top of your shoulders toward your ears.
Keep your head and neck straight.

　両肩の先を両耳まで持ち上げる。頭と首はまっすぐにする

Relax shoulders downward into normal position.

　肩の力を抜いて元の位置まで下ろす

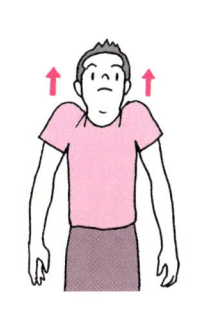

Bring your right shoulder up to the right earlobe.

　右肩を右の耳たぶまで上げる

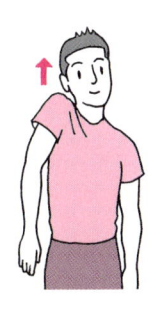

Support your right elbow with your left hand.

　右肘を左手で支える

With your left hand pull your right elbow across your chest.

　左手で右肘を胸の前を横切るように引っ張る

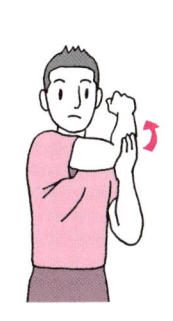

section 4 Passive ROM Exercise
他動的関節可動域訓練

ROM=Range of Motion

I'm going to grasp your palm.
掌を握りますよ

Your forearm is supported at the wrist with my hand.
手首のところで前腕を支えます

Forearm is bent upward.
前腕を上方に曲げます

Elbow and upper arm are flat on the table.
肘と二の腕は台の上に平らに置きます

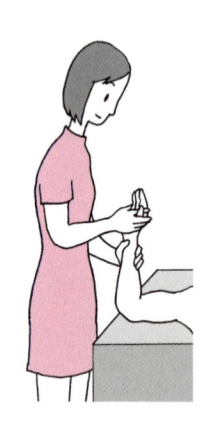

The hand is bent forward at the wrist.
手を手首のところで前のほうに曲げます

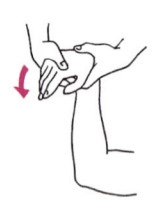

The hand is stretched backward from the wrist.
手を手首のところで後ろのほうへ伸ばします

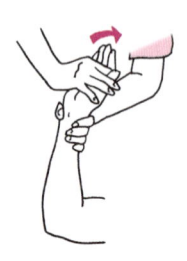

Move to ulnar side.
(The hand is bent toward the side of the little finger.)
 尺骨のほうへ動かします
 （手を小指のほうへ曲げます）

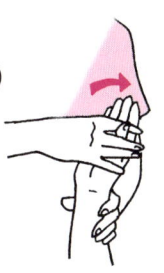

Move to radial side.
(The hand is bent toward the thumb.)
 橈骨のほうへ動かします
 （手を親指のほうへ曲げます）

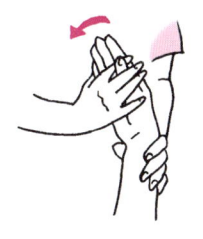

section 5 Muscle Test : Upper Body
筋力測定評価：上半身

肘関節：屈曲

Make a fist.
Keep your arms straight in front of you.
　げんこつをつくって、両腕を前にまっすぐ伸ばしてください

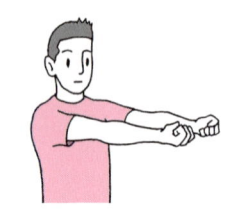

Bend your arms toward your shoulders.
Try to strengthen your bent elbow.
　両腕を肩のほうに曲げて。曲げた肘に力を入れてください

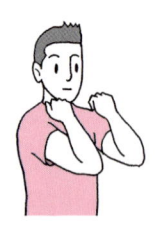

I will grasp your elbow and your wrist and try to pull your forearm down. Resist my pulling.
　肘と手首をつかんで、前腕を下に引きますよ。引っ張られないよう抵抗してください

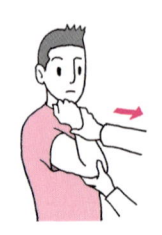

Rest your elbow and forearm on the table.
Make a fist.
　　肘と前腕を台に乗せて。げんこつをつくってください
Move your forearm toward your chest.
　　前腕を自分の胸のほうに動かしてください

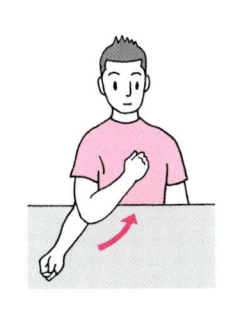

肘関節：伸展

I will grasp your wrist and upper arm just above the elbow.
　　手首と上腕の肘のすぐ上のところをつかみますよ
Keep your palms down.
I will push your forearm down.
　　手のひらを下に向けてください。前腕を押し下げますよ
Resist my pushing.
　　押されないよう抵抗してください

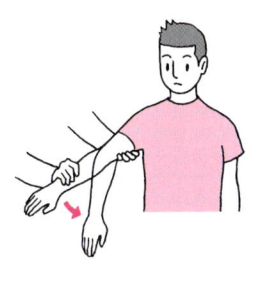

二頭筋

Hold your arm in front of you with the elbow bent.
　　肘を曲げて腕を前に出してください
I will grasp your wrist and try to pull your forearm down, while pushing against your upper arm. Resist my pulling.
　　あなたの手首をつかんで前腕を下に引きます。その間、
　　二の腕を押します。腕が下がらないよう抵抗してください

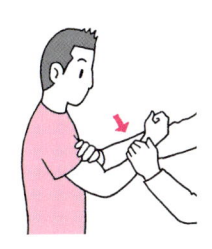

section5 Muscle Test : Upper Body　筋力測定評価：上半身

上腕三頭筋 (Triceps Brachii)

I will grasp your wrist and try to push your forearm upward.
　あなたの手首を握って前腕を上方に押します
Try to strengthen your arm and resist my pushing.
　腕に力をこめて押されないよう抵抗してください

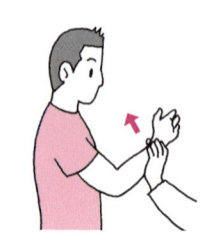

腕・肩 (Arm, Shoulder)

Hold your arms out straight in front of you, palms facing.
　腕をまっすぐ前に伸ばして、両手のひらが向き合うようにしてください
I will try to separate your arms. Resist my pressure.
　両腕を離しますから、私の力に抵抗してください

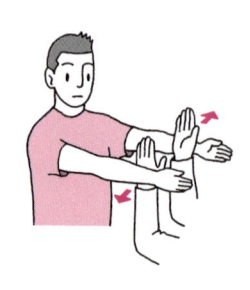

Extend arms palms up.
　手のひらを上に向けて両腕をまっすぐ伸ばしてください。
Maintain the same level.
Hold this position for 30 seconds.
　同じ高さを保って、そのまま30秒間じっとしていてください

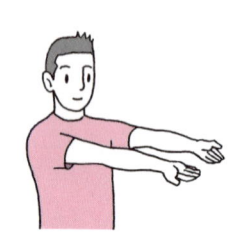

If one arm lowers, your shoulder girdle is weak on that side.
　片方の腕が下がるようですと、そちら側の肩甲帯が弱っているのです

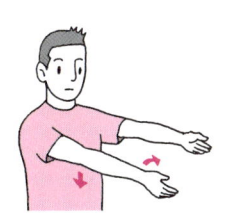

I will place my hands on your forearms.
　あなたの前腕に私の両手を置きます
I will apply downward pressure.
Try to resist my pressure.
　下に向けて押しますので、押されないよう抵抗してください

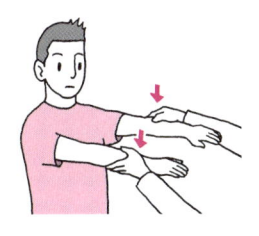

Stretch your arms out to your sides shoulder level. Palms down.
　両腕を伸ばして肩の高さにしてください。手のひらは下向きです

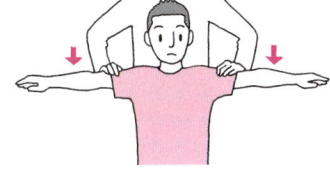

I will try to press your upper arms down.
Resist my pressure.
　あなたの両腕を押し下げます。私の力に抵抗してください

section5 Muscle Test : Upper Body　筋力測定評価：上半身

Sit down in front of me.
　私の前に座ってください

I will place my hands on your shoulders.
　あなたの両肩に私の両手を置きます

Try to raise your shoulders as I press them down.
　私は両肩を押し下げますから、あなたは押し上げてください

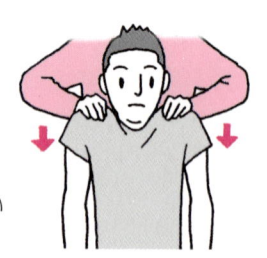

手首（Wrist）

I will grasp your forearm just above the wrist. Make a fist.
　前腕の手首のすぐ上を握りますよ。げんこつをつくってください

I will try to push your hand upward with my fist. Resist my pressure.
　私のこぶしであなたの手を押し上げます。押されないよう抵抗してください

Try to push your hand backward against my fist.
　私の握りこぶしをあなたの手で甲側に押し返してください

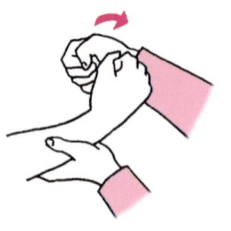

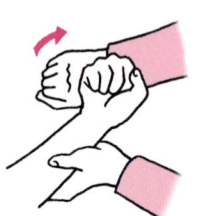

握力測定 (Handgrip strength)

I will extend my first and second fingers.
Grasp my fingers and squeeze......... Let them go.
> 人差し指と中指を出しますから、2本の指を握って締め付けてください……では指を離してください

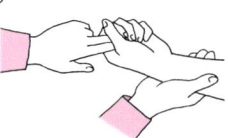

親指とそれ以外の指 (Thumb, Fingers)

Grasp the edge of the paper between your thumb and other fingers.
> 親指と残りの4本の指で紙の端をつかんでください

Pull the paper toward you, resisting my counter-pulling.
> 自分のほうに紙を引っ張ってください。私は逆方向に引っ張りますから

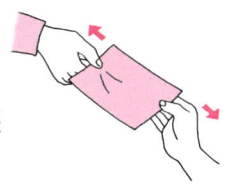

Grasp the paper with your index finger and thumb, hand upward.
> 人差し指と親指で紙をつかみ、手首を立ててください

Resist my pulling, alternating your grasp with your other fingers and thumb one by one.
> 指を1本ずつ変えながら親指とで紙をはさみ、私に引っ張られないようしてください

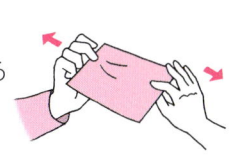

section5 Muscle Test : Upper Body　筋力測定評価：上半身

Make a ring with your thumb and index finger.
　親指と人差し指で輪を作ってください

I will try to hook my index finger in your ring and pull it toward myself. Resist my pulling.
　その輪に人差し指を引っ掛けて、私のほうに引っ張りますから抵抗してください

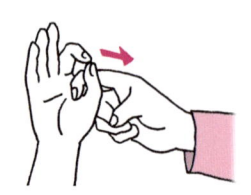

section 6 Muscle Test : Lower Body
筋力測定評価：下半身

脚

Lie prone. Keep your thighs flat on the floor.
うつぶせになって、太腿を平らにして床につけてください

Raise both legs to the same height.
両脚を同じ高さまで上げてください

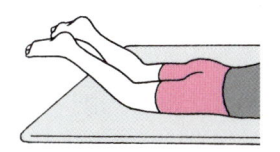

If one leg lowers, there is a weakness in that leg.
片方の脚が下がるようですと、そちら側の脚が弱いのです

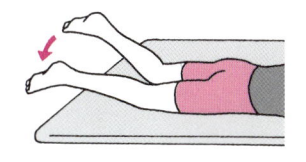

膝

Sit at the side of the table, legs dangling.
両脚をぶらぶらさせて台の端に座ってください

Try to raise your thigh as I press down on your knee.
私は膝を押し下げますから、あなたは太腿を持ち上げてください

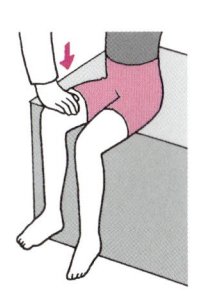

section6 Muscle Test : Lower Body　筋力測定評価：下半身

I will place my hand on your knee and your lower leg.
　私の手をあなたの膝と膝下のところに当てます

I will try to pull your leg outward.
Resist my pressure.
　あなたの足をこちら側に引きますから、私の力に抵抗して
　ください

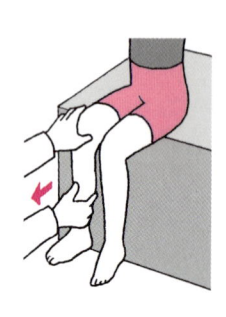

足

I will grab your ankle and push your toes back.
Resist my pushing.
　あなたの足首を握って足指をそらします。
　押し返してください

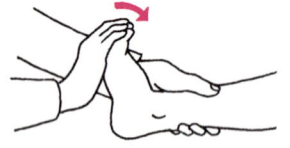

I will grasp your heel and try to pull your foot downward. Resist my pulling.
　あなたの踵を握って足を下向きに引きます。引っ張られな
　いよう抵抗してください

PART 2　病院の中での運動・動作表現

Extend your feet over the end of the bed.
　ベッドの端から両脚を出してください

I will press against the sole of your foot with my hand. So, push against my hand.
　私の手で足の裏を押しますから、押し返してください

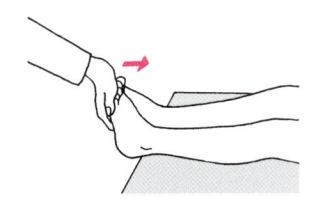

I will hold the middle of your foot.
　足の真ん中あたりをつかみますよ

Try to pull your foot up toward your knee, while I am trying to hold it down.
　足を膝のほうへそらしてください。
　その間、私は下向けに引きます

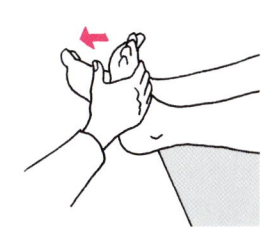

section 7 Functional Assessments
さまざまな機能検査

平衡機能：片脚立ち（Equilibrium : Standing on one foot）

① Stand straight with both feet together.
Arms extended at your sides.
両足をそろえて、まっすぐに立ってください。
両腕は脇につけて伸ばします

② Stand with one leg in front of the other.
片方の脚を前に出して立ってください

③ Bend one knee, thigh forward and foot back.
Try to maintain that position.
片膝を曲げて太腿を前に出し、足は後ろに引いてください。そのままの姿勢を保ってください

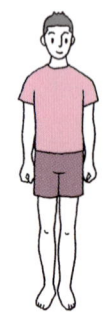

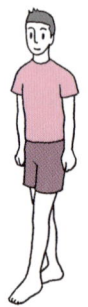

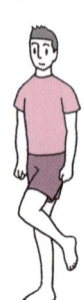

PART 2　病院の中での運動・動作表現

踵膝試験（Heel-toe test）

① Lie with legs extended. Raise one leg.
両脚を伸ばして横になり、片脚を上げてください

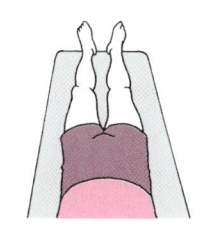

② Bend your knee and top your heel to your opposite knee.
膝を曲げて踵を反対側の膝に乗せてください

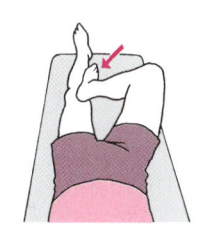

③ Straighten that leg.
Do the same with the other leg.
その脚をまっすぐに伸ばします。
もう一方の脚でも同様にしてください

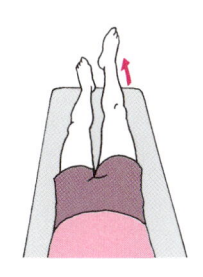

section7 Functional Assessments　さまざまな機能検査

膝蓋腱反射 (Patellar tendon reflex)

① Could you flex your knee to 90 degrees?
　膝を90度に曲げてください

② I will palpate the patellar tendon with a reflex hammer.
　膝蓋腱反射用ハンマーで触れます

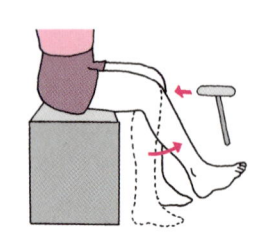

急速変換試験 (Diadochokinetic test : Working in turn)

① Sit with both feet flat on the floor. Rest your hands palms up on the knees.
　両足を平らに床につけて座ってください。
　両手のひらを上向きにして両膝に乗せてください

② Tap your knees alternately palm up and palms down. Do it quickly.
　手の甲と手のひらで交互に膝を打ってください。
　すばやくこの動作をおこないます

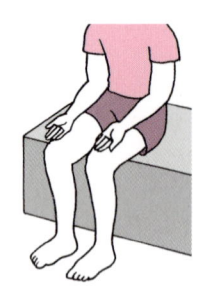

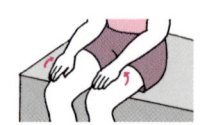

外輪筋検査＝眼球を動かす筋肉のアセスメント

(Test of Extraocular muscle ＝ Assessment of eye muscle Function)

Look straight ahead.
まっすぐ前を向いて

Remain still. Don't move your head.
じっとして頭を動かさないで

① Watch my index finger at a distance of about 50cm in front of your nose.
鼻先50センチのところにある私の人差し指を見てください

② Follow the movement of my finger with your eyes without moving your head.
頭を動かさずに目で私の指の動きを追ってください

③ From the midline to your right side.
正中線からあなたの右側に動きます

④ Upward, staying to the right of the midline.
右位置のままで上方に動きます

⑤ Downward, staying to the right of the midline.
右位置のまま下方に動きます

⑥ Left, across the midline.
正中線を横切って左側に行きます

⑦ Upward staying to the left of the midline.
左位置のまま上方に行きます

⑧ Straight down, staying to the left of the midline.
左位置のまままっすぐ下方に動きます

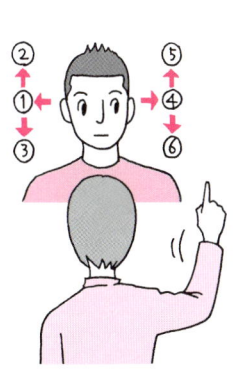

section7 Functional Assessments　さまざまな機能検査

小脳機能：指鼻試験（Cerebellum Function : Finger-Nose test）

① Touch your nose with your index finger of your right hand.
　右手の人差し指で自分の鼻に触れてください

② Pull it away. Do the same with your left hand, alternating each hand.
　その指を離してください。左手でも同じことをしてください。手を変えて交互に

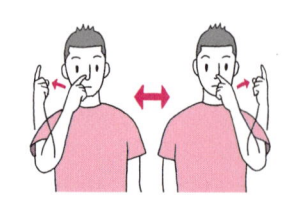

① Touch my index finger with yours.
　あなたの人差し指で私の人差し指を触ってください

② Then bring your finger to your nose, alternating between my index finger and your nose.
　その指を自分の鼻にもっていきます。
　私の人差し指と自分の鼻とを交互に触れてください

③ I will move my finger away. Try to continue to touch my finger and your nose alternately.
　私の指をずらして動かしていきます。そのまま続けて
　私の指とあなたの鼻を交互に触ってください

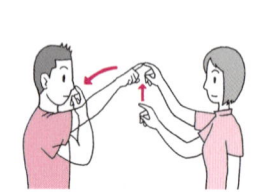

PART 2　病院の中での運動・動作表現

対立運動 (Opposition exercise)

Touch the little finger and thumb together.
親指と小指を触れ合わせてください

Touch the four fingers to the thumb one by one.
親指とそれぞれの指を触れ合わせてください

Fold your thumb and touch the base of your little finger.
親指を曲げて小指のつけ根に触れてください

Repeat this four times.
4回繰り返してください

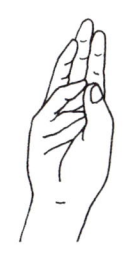

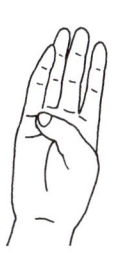

指の運動 (Finger Motion)

Rotate your thumbs around each other.
親指同士をくるくる回してください

Rotate index fingers, middle fingers, medical fingers, and little fingers, around each other.
人差し指同士、中指同士、薬指同士、小指同士をくるくる回してください

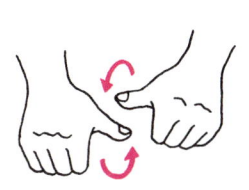

section7 Functional Assessments　さまざまな機能検査

肩の旋回（Shoulder Rotation）

With bent elbow and open palm.
肘を曲げ手のひらを開いた状態にします

The forearm is raised and lowered, which twists the upper arm.
前腕を上下させることで、上腕をひねります

This results in shoulder rotation.
これで肩を回したことになります

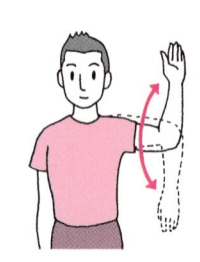

股関節可動域（Hip Joint ROM）

① Sit at the edge of the table, knees apart. Press the soles of both feet together.
膝を開いて台の端に座って。両方の足裏をぴったり合わせてください

Allow your arms to dangle freely, palms up.
両腕はだらりと下げ、手のひらを上に向けます

② Holding that position, rotate your head from side to side.
そのままの姿勢で首を左右に回してください

③ Holding that position, press your chin to your chest.
そのままの姿勢であごを胸につけてください

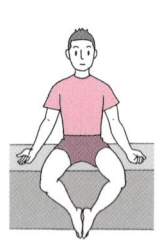

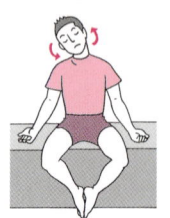

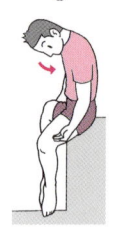

顎関節可動域（Temporomandibular Joint ROM）

I will place my fingers into the temples.
私の両方の指をあなたのこめかみにおきます

Open and close your mouth.
口を開けたり閉じたりしてください

Let your jaw up and down.
顎を上げたり下げたりしてください

Then, protract and retract your mandible.
次に下顎を突き出したり、引っ込めたりしてください

Move your lower teeth (lower jaw) laterally.
下の歯（下顎）を左右に動かしてください

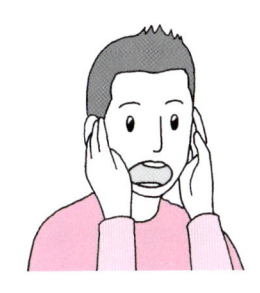

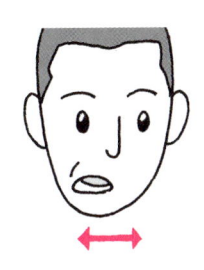

section 8 Diagnostic Tests
さまざまな診断検査

血液検査（Blood test）

I'll take a blood sample.
採血をします

Roll up your sleeve and extend your arm.
袖をまくって腕を伸ばしてください

I'll apply a tourniquet.
腕に駆血帯を巻きます

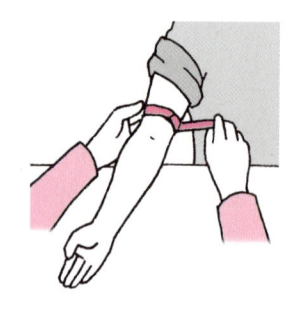

Make a fist.
手のひらを握ってください

Extend your fingers.
では、手のひらを開いてください

Lightly press the alcohol swab to the needle site.
アルコール綿を上から軽く指で押さえてください

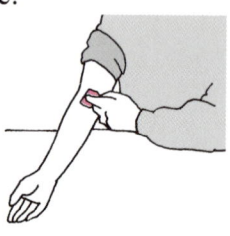

PART 2　病院の中での運動・動作表現

X線検査やMR検査の場面（X-ray examination & MRI test）

Remove your clothes and put on this gown.
この検査着に着替えてください

Remove all metal items, wrist watch and jewelries.
時計やアクセサリーなど金属製のものはすべてはずしてください

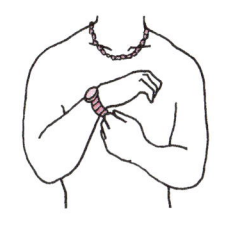

Go into room Five.
5番の部屋に入ってください

Lie on your back (right side).
台の上に仰向け（右を下にして）に寝てください

Put your chin on the chin-rest.
あごをカセットの上に乗せてください

Put your arms around the auto cassette.
両腕で自動カセッテを抱くようにしてください

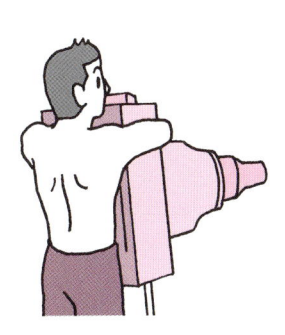

071

section8 Diagnostic Tests　さまざまな診断検査

Take a deep breath.　Hold.
　大きく息を吸って、止めてください

Expand your abdomen. (Draw in your abdomen.)
　おなかをふくらませてください（ひっこめてください）

Swallow the contents of the cup in one gulp.
　コップの中身を一気に飲んでください

Please call me if you feel unwell.
　具合が悪くなったら声をかけてください

診察場面 (Consultation)

I'll listen to your heart with a stethoscope.
Please lift your top and bare your chest.
　聴診器をあてます。洋服を上げて胸を出してください

Turn around and show me your back.
　後ろを向いて、背中を出してください

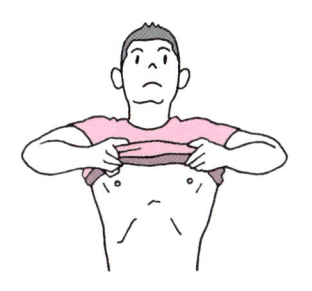

I'll check your throat.
Open your mouth wide.
　喉をみますので、口を大きく開けてください

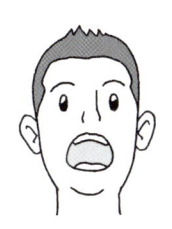

Stick out your tongue.
　舌を出してみてください

section8 Diagnostic Tests　さまざまな診断検査

心電図検査（Electrocardiogram=ECG）

Pull your socks down below your ankles.
靴下を下げて足首を出してください

Please strip to your waist.
上半身裸になってください

I'm going to attach some electrodes to your chest.
胸にいくつか電極をつけます

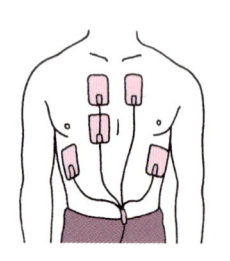

呼吸機能検査（Examination of the respiratory system）

Take a deep breath.
息を深く吸ってください

Hold your breath for 10 seconds.
１０秒間、息を止めてください

Breathe out, all at once.
勢いよく全部吐き出してください

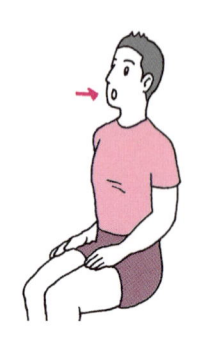

脳波検査 (EEG examination)

Close your eyes and relax.
目を閉じて楽にしてください

A light will flash in front of your eyes.
目の前で光が点滅します

Keep your eyes closed.
目を閉じたままにして

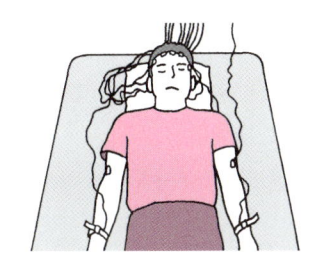

超音波テスト (Ultrasound)

I'm going to put jelly on your abdomen.
おなかにゼリーを塗ります

Sit up and turn your body to the right.
体を起こして右に向けてください

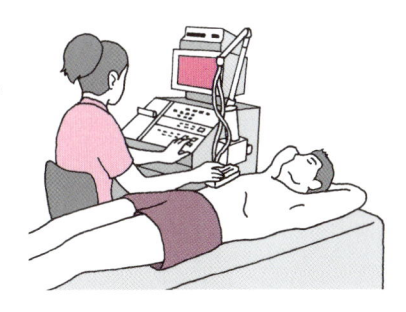

section 9 Positioning
体位

Semi-prone position　半腹臥位

Lie on a side with a pillow between arms for support. Your face is turned to one side.
　両腕に枕をはさんで体の支えとし、横向けに寝ます。
　顔は横向きです

This is for mucus discharge from the back lobes.
　後背部の痰を排出するための体位です

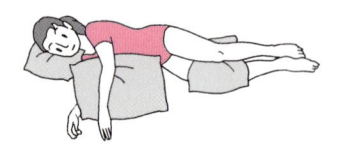

Semi-supine position　半背臥位

Take a back-lying position with body turned to 45-degree.
　体を45度に傾けて仰向けになってください

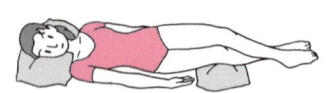

Supine position　背臥位（仰臥位）

Lie on your back with the largest area providing the base of support.
　基底面積が最も広くなるよう仰向けに寝ます
This way, you can keep a low center of gravity.
　重心が低い姿勢です

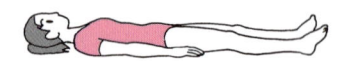

PART 2　病院の中での運動・動作表現

Lateral position　側臥位

Take a side-lying position with body turned to 90 degrees. Keep your leg slightly flexed.
　体を90度にして横向きに寝てください。軽く足を曲げています
This is for passing duodenal drainage tube.
　十二指腸ドレナージ挿管のための体位です

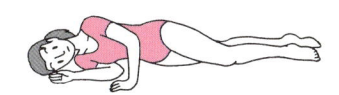

Prone position　腹臥位（伏臥位）

Lie down on the abdomen. Your face is turned to one side to prevent inhalation of vomitus.
　うつ伏せに寝てください。吐瀉物を飲み込まないよう
　顔は横向きです

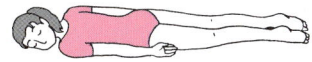

Sims's position　シムス位

Take a face-lying position on the pillow with body pressure removed from the buttocks.
　枕の上にうつ伏せに寝てお尻の力を抜きます
Knee and thigh are drawn upward toward the chest.
　膝と腿を胸のほうへ引き寄せます
This is a comfortable resting position.
　楽な休息の姿勢です

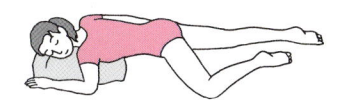

section9 Positioning　体位

Trendelenburg position　骨盤高位, トレンデレンブルグ位

Your head is low, and body and legs are on an elevated and inclined plane.

　頭は低くして、胴体と両脚を上向きの斜面に乗せてください

This is for pelvic or abdominal surgery.

　骨盤や腹部の手術のためです

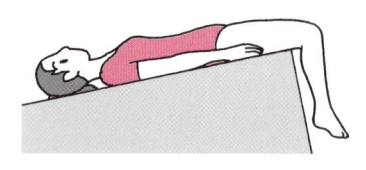

Fowler's position　半座位, ファーラー位

The head of the bed is elevated. It inclines 45 to 60 degrees from horizontal. The knees can either be bent or straight.

　ベッドの頭の部分を上げます。45度から60度の傾斜
　にします。膝は曲げても、伸ばしたままでもかまいません

This position facilitates breathing.

　こうすると呼吸が楽になります

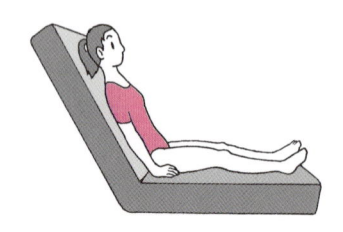

Lithotomy position 載石位

Raise and open both hips and legs with bent knees.
　膝を曲げて両股関節と両脚を上げ、開いてください

Thighs are rotated externally.
　大腿を外向きに回します

This is for diagnosis and treatment of uterus.
　子宮の診断および治療のための体位です

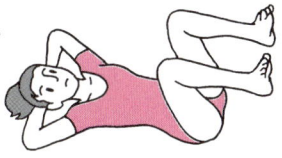

Knee-chest position (genupectoral position) 膝胸位

Kneel down. Your body is supported by the knees and chest.
　ひざまずいて、身体を両膝と胸で支えます

Stick out the buttocks with head on the floor.
　頭を床につけて、お尻を突き出してください

This is a posture to correct bleach position of fetus.
　逆子を矯正するための姿勢です

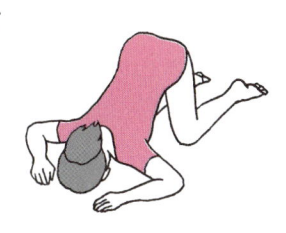

section9 Positioning　体位

Long sitting position　長座位

Sit with legs extended. Keep tension in the upper torso.

両足を伸ばして座ってください。上半身は緊張させて

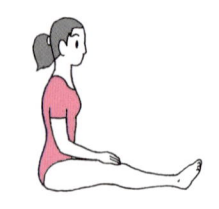

Agura（Sitting cross-legged）　あぐら

Sit with both knees flexed, legs crossed. The center of gravity is low.

両膝を曲げて両足を交差させて座ってください。重心は低くなっています

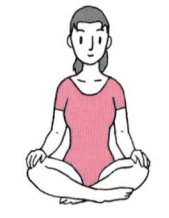

Japanese sitting　正座

Kneel with hips resting on the heels.

両踵にお尻を乗せて両膝をついて座ります

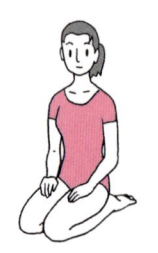

Orthopneic position　起座位

Sit on a chair with your head resting on a pillow. Arms supported on a table. The upper trunk is nearly upright, a little bent forward, position.

枕の上に頭を乗せて椅子に座ってください。両腕を台で支えてください。上半身はほぼまっすぐ、やや前傾です。

This allows ease of breathing when heart or pulmonary condition is poor.

肺や心臓が弱っているときに呼吸が楽になります

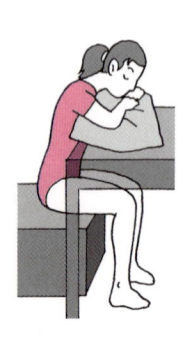

Chair-sitting　椅座位

Sit on a chair with back straight.
Feet are flat on the floor.
　背中をまっすぐにして椅子に座ってください。
　両足は床に平らにつけます

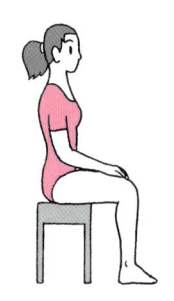

Chair-straddling　椅子にまたがる姿勢

Sit straddling a chair.
　椅子にまたがって座ってください
This position is for thoracentesis.
　胸腔穿刺のための姿勢です

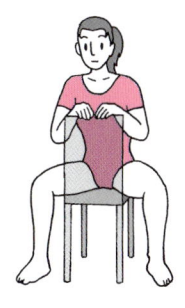

Forward-leaning sitting　前傾座位

Sit on a chair leaning forward.
　体を前向きに傾けて椅子に座ってください

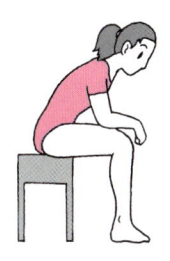

付録
関節可動域運動の専門的な表現と一般的な表現

Professional | Lay

専門表現 　　図解 　　　　　　　　　　　　　　　患者向け表現

neck 首・頸

Professional	Lay
頸の屈曲（前屈） Neck flexion 頸椎屈曲を行う Flex cervical spine.	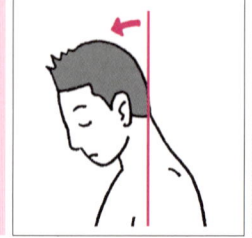 首（頭）を前に倒す Forward bent position of neck/ head 首を下に向けて（顎をひいて）ください Keep your neck and head bent forward. (Chin points to your chest.)
頸の伸展（後屈） Neck extension 頸椎伸展を行う Extend cervical spine. 頸の過伸展 Neck hyperextension 頸の過伸展を行う Cervical spine is hyperextended.	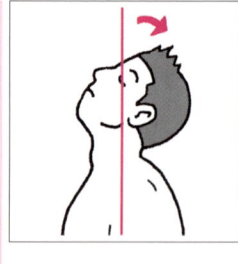 首（頭）を後ろに倒す Back tilt of head Tilt your head backward. 首（頭）をずっと後ろに倒してください Far-backward tilt of head 頭をずっと後方に伸ばしてください Keep your head and neck bent far back.
頸の回旋 Neck rotation 頸を回旋させる Rotate cervical spine.	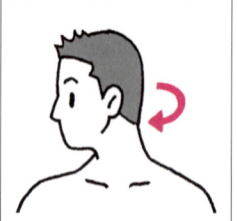 首を横に向ける Side turn of head 顔を肩のほうに回してください Turn your head to one side toward the shoulder. 次に円を描くように頭を回してください Then, turn head in circular motion.
頸の側屈 Lateral flexion of neck 頸を側方に屈曲させる Flex neck laterally.	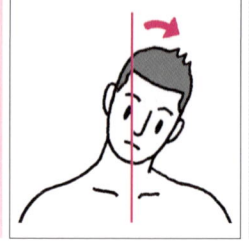 頭を横に倒す Sideway tilt of head 頭を片方に倒してください Tilt your head down to one side. できる限り倒してください Tilt as far as possible.

付録　関節可動域運動の専門的な表現と一般的な表現

Professional
専門表現　　　図解

Lay
患者向け表現

shoulder　肩

専門表現	図解	患者向け表現
肩甲帯の屈曲・伸展 Shoulder flexion/extension	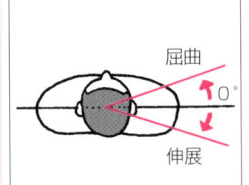 屈曲 0° 伸展	肩を前に（後ろに）動かしてください Rotate your shoulder forward and then rotate it backward.
肩甲帯の挙上・引き下げ（下制） Shoulder elevation/depression	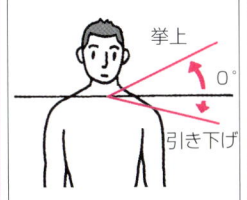 挙上 0° 引き下げ	肩を上に上げてください。下に下げてください Raise and lower your shoulders.
肩の外旋・内旋 External/Internal rotation of shoulder	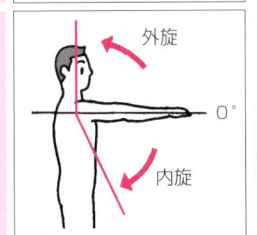 外旋 0° 内旋	腕を前に水平に出し、頭上に上げてください。次に脇まで下ろしてください Extend both arms horizontally, straight ahead. Raise your arms above your head. Then, lower your arms to your sides.
肩の内転 Shoulder adduction	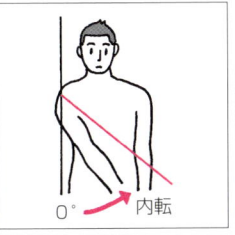 0° 内転	体の横に下ろした腕を体の内側にもっていきます。もう一方の腕も同様にします Keep your arms down to your sides. Cross your straightened arm to your opposite side in front of you. Then do the same with your opposite arm.
肩の側方挙上・内転 Shoulder abduction/adduction	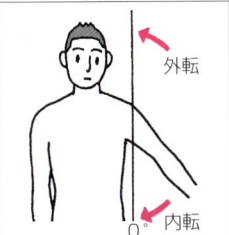 外転 0° 内転	腕を体の脇につけ、横に開いてください。元に戻してください Extend your arm sideways and up, as far as possible. Return to a starting position.

085

Professional	図解	Lay 患者向け表現
肩の前方挙上・後方挙上 Forward flexion of shoulder/ Backward extension of shoulder	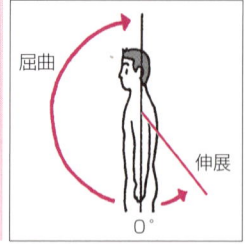 屈曲／伸展 0°	脇に下ろした腕をまっすぐ前方に上げてください。元に戻して、今度はまっすぐ後ろに引いてください Your arms are at your sides. Raise your extended arm forward. Lower it to the starting position. Then, pull your extended arm backward, behind body.
肩の水平屈曲・水平伸展 Horizontal flexion (adduction) of shoulder Horizontal extension (abduction) of shoulder	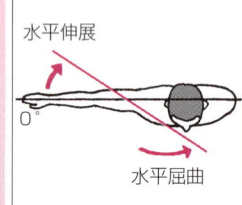 水平伸展／水平屈曲 0°	腕を肩の高さまで水平に上げ、手の甲は下に向けます。腕をまっすぐにしたまま体の前のほうへもっていきます。次に背中のほうへもっていきます Raise your arm to a horizontal position shoulder height. With arm extended, bring it toward the center, palm down. Then, extend your arm backward toward your back.

arm　腕

Professional	図解	Lay
肘の屈曲・伸展 Elbow flexion/ extension	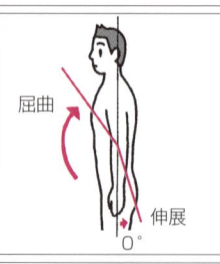 屈曲／伸展 0°	脇につけた肘を曲げて前腕を前方にもっていきます。元に戻して、今度は肘を伸ばして腕を後ろにもっていきます Bring your forearm upward, elbow bent at your side. Return to starting position. Then, pull your forearm backward, elbow locked.
右肘は軽く屈曲 Right elbow partially flexed.		右肘を軽く曲げてください Bend slightly your right elbow.
両肘とも屈曲 Both elbows are flexed.		両腕を曲げてください Bend your elbows.

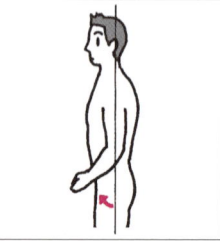

付録　関節可動域運動の専門的な表現と一般的な表現

Professional
専門表現　　　図解

Lay
患者向け表現

専門表現	図解	患者向け表現
左肘は伸展 Left elbow is extended.		左肘を伸ばしてください Straighten your left elbow.
前腕の回内・回外 Forearm pronation/supination	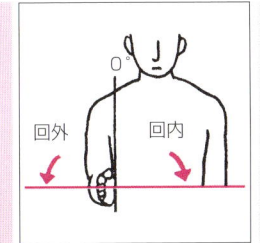	前腕を肘のところで90度に曲げ、手のひらだけを床に向けたり、天井に向けたりしてください Bend your forearm at the elbow bringing your forearm to form an L-shape position. Then rotate your hand palm facing up, then, palm facing down. Do not move elbow or shoulder.

hand, finger　手・指

専門表現	図解	患者向け表現
手の屈曲（掌屈）・伸展（背屈） Hand flexion (palmarfexion)/ Hand extension (dorsiflexion)	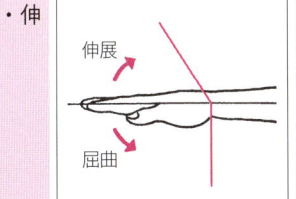	手のひらを床に向け、手首を上下に動かしてください Palm facing down, move plam toward inner aspect of forearm (flexion). Bend your hand at the wrist pulling your hand up and back (extention).
手の橈屈・尺屈 Radial deviation/ Ulnar deviation	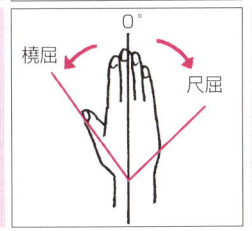	手のひらを床に向け、手首を左右に動かしてください Palm facing down, rotate your hand toward your thumb and then, toward your little finger.
指の外転 Fingers abduction.	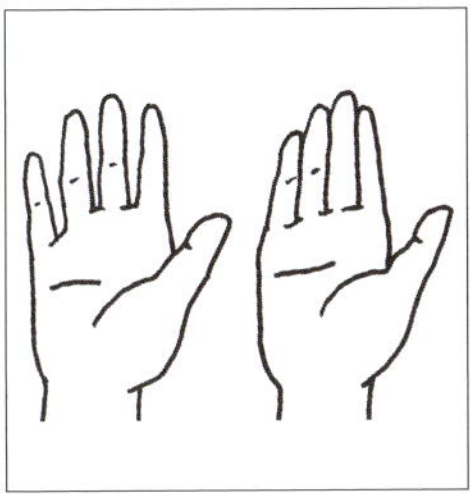	指を開く Fingers are spread apart.
指の内転 Fingers adduction.		指を閉じる Fingers are brought together.

Professional 専門表現	図解	Lay 患者向け表現
指の伸展 Fingers extension.	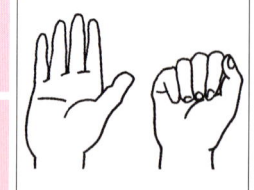	指をまっすぐ伸ばす Fingers are stretched straight apart.
指の屈曲 Fingers flexion		指を曲げる Fingers are bent onto the palm.
親指の外転・内転 Thumb abduction. Thumb adduction	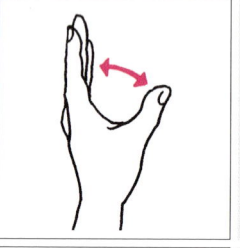	親指を人差し指から離す Extend your thumb out away from your index finger. 親指を人差し指に近づける Position your thumb next to the index finger
小指へのオポジション Opposition to little finger. 親指の伸展・屈曲 Thumb extension/flexion.	Opposition to little finger / Extension flexion	親指を小指のほうへもっていく Move the thumb across the palm to touch the little finger. 親指を掌に近づける・掌から離す Bend the thumb into the palm. Then, position the thumb away from the palm.

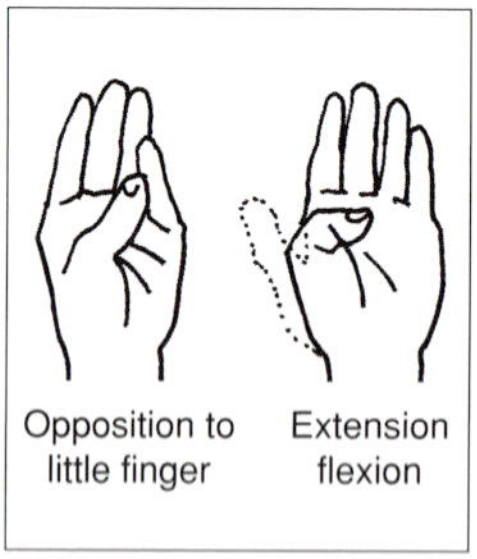

thoracic & lumbar 胸腰部 / body (trunk) 胸腰部

全運動範囲を通じて胸部を骨盤のほうへ屈曲 Patient flexes thorax on pelvis through range of motion.	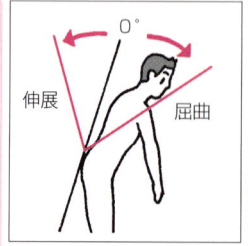 0° 伸展 屈曲	上半身を起こし、腰から上体をそらす Raise your upper body and bend yourself backward as much as possible. 次に前方に曲げる Then bend yourself forward as much as possible.

付録　関節可動域運動の専門的な表現と一般的な表現

Professional
専門表現　　　　　図解

Lay
患者向け表現

専門表現	図解	患者向け表現
胸腰部の右側屈, 左側屈 Lateral bending of thorax and lumber	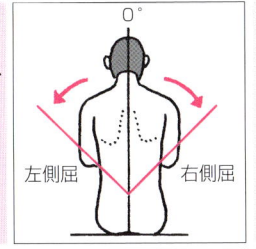	上体を起こし、右に傾ける，左に傾ける Raise your upper torso, tilt it to right side. Then, to the left side.
胸郭の左回旋, 右回旋 Rotation of thorax to left. Rotation of thorax to right.	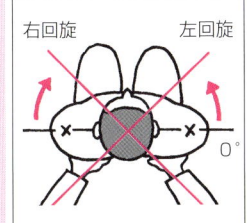	上半身を左に回す Rotate your upper torso to the left. 上半身を右に回す Rotation your upper torso to the right.
脊椎の屈曲・伸展 Flexion of spine Extension of spine	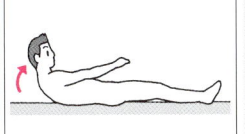 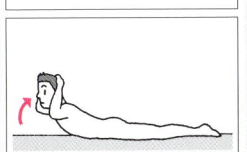	仰向けになり，両腕を足のほうに延ばして上半身を起こす From a back lying position, the upper body is raised upward with arms stretched toward the feet. うつ伏せになり，両手を頭の後ろで組んで上半身を高く持ち上げる Lying on the abdomen, the upper body is raised upward to a high position with hands clasped behind the head.

Professional | Lay
専門表現　　　図解　　　　　　　患者向け表現

pelvis / hips　骨盤・殿部

Professional		Lay
殿部の内転・外転 Hip abduction Hip adduction	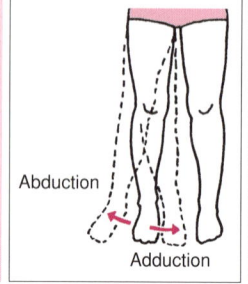 *Abduction / Adduction illustration*	脚を股関節のところで中央から外側に伸ばす Your leg is pulled away from the body center at the hip. 脚を中央に戻して今度は内側に伸ばす Bring your leg toward the body center. Cross it toward the opposite side.
内旋・外旋 Inward rotation Outward rotation	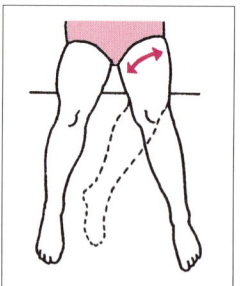 *Inward/outward rotation illustration*	脚を股関節のところで内側に回す Roll your leg inward at the hip joint. 脚を股関節のところで外側に回す Roll your leg outward at the hip joint.
内旋・外旋 Inward/ outward rotation	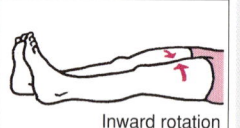 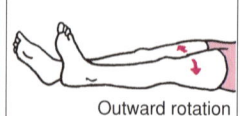 *Inward rotation / Outward rotation illustration*	脚をまっすぐ伸ばし内側そして外側に回転させる Your stretched legs are rolled inward and outward at the hips and thighs.
殿部の屈曲・伸展 Hip flexion Hip extension	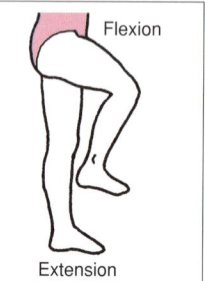 *Flexion / Extension illustration*	膝を曲げて脚をお尻までもち上げる Your knee is bent and leg is raised upward at the hip. もう一方の脚はまっすぐ伸ばしたままにする You other leg remains straight from the hip.

付録　関節可動域運動の専門的な表現と一般的な表現

Professional
専門表現　　　　図解

Lay
患者向け表現

専門表現	患者向け表現
殿部の過伸展 Hip hyperextension	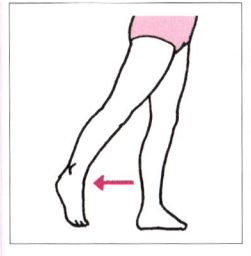 膝をまっすぐ伸ばしたまま片方の脚をできるだけ後ろに引く One leg is stretched far backward from the hip with a straight knee.

leg・knee　脚・膝

専門表現	患者向け表現
長座位 Long-sitting 下肢は骨盤に対して垂直位 Legs are in vertical alignment with pelvis.	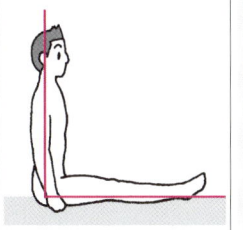 体重を均等にかけて骨盤と両脚が直角になるようにする Keep your weight evenly balanced so that your pelvis and legs are in straight line.
膝の屈曲・伸展 Knee flexion Knee extension	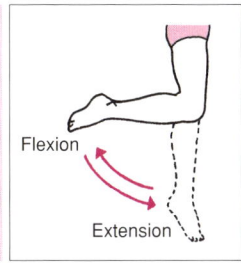 脚を膝から後方に上げる Your leg is raised backward from the knee. もう一方の脚と膝はまっすぐにする Your other leg and knee is straight.
回旋足動 Circumduction	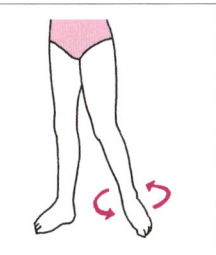 円を描くように足を回す Move leg in circle.

091

Professional / Lay

専門表現　　　図解　　　　　　　　　　　患者向け表現

foot　足

Professional	Lay
足は下腿に対し直角 Foot is at right angle to the leg	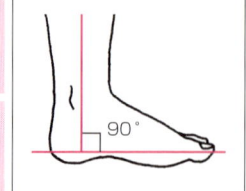 足と脚を90度に保つ The angle of your foot and leg should be 90 degrees.
足は軽く外反 Foot has slight eversion.	足を軽く外に向ける Your foot slightly points outward.
回外 Supination	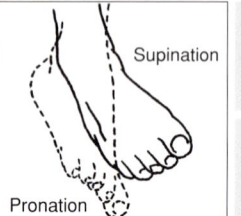 足を足首のところで内側に回してください Rotate your foot inward at the ankle. Pull your foot inward.
回内 Pronation	足を足首のところで外側に向けてください Rotate your foot outward at the ankle.
背側屈曲 Dorsal flexion	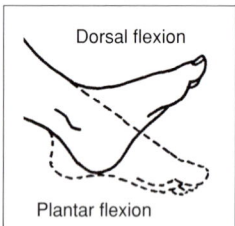 足を上に向けます Your foot is pointing up.
足底屈曲 Plantar flexion	足を下へ向けます Your foot is pointing down.
つま先の屈曲・伸展 Toe flexion Toe extension	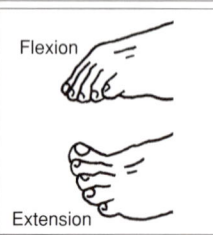 つま先を下方に曲げる Your toes are bent downward. つま先を上方にそらす Your toes are pulled upward.
つま先の外転・内転 Toe adduction Toe abduction	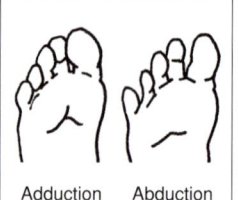 足の指をくっつける Your toes are all together. 足の指を離す Your toes spread apart.